The Side Crunch Solution

Pain-Free, Effective Core Training from Head to Toe

Helen Talbott

Disclaimer

The information contained in this book is for educational and informational purposes only and is not intended to be a substitute for professional medical advice, diagnosis, or treatment. Always consult with a qualified healthcare professional before starting any new exercise program, especially if you have any pre-existing medical conditions or injuries.

The author and publisher of this book do not claim to guarantee any specific results or outcomes from using the information or exercises provided. Individual results may vary depending on a variety of factors, including individual health, fitness level, and consistency of practice.

The exercises and techniques described in this book should be performed with caution and proper form. It is the reader's responsibility to ensure their safety and to adjust or modify the exercises as needed based on their own physical limitations and abilities.

Table of contents

About the author

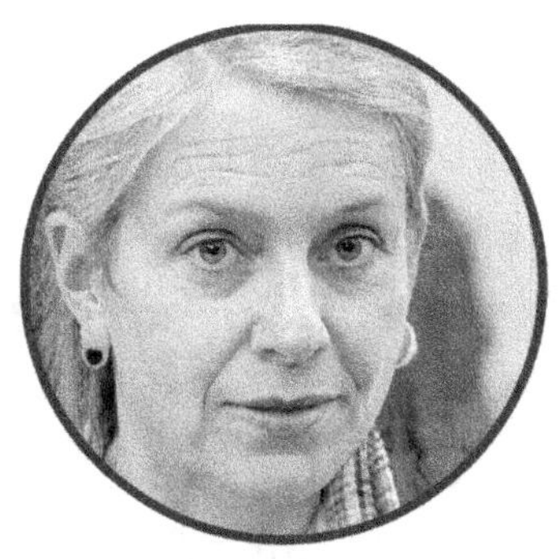

Helen Talbott, the author of "The Side Crunch Solution: Pain-Free, Effective Core Training from Head to Toe," isn't just a fitness enthusiast; she's a passionate advocate for core health and functional movement. Her journey began with a personal quest to overcome chronic back pain, leading her to discover the transformative power of side crunches and their impact on core stability and overall well-being.

Driven by this revelation, Helen embarked on a mission to share her knowledge and empower others to unlock the potential of their core. Through extensive research, collaboration with fitness professionals, and countless hours of refining her approach, she developed a holistic system focused on pain-free, effective core training with side crunches as the cornerstone.

Helen's expertise extends beyond traditional exercise science. With a background in [insert relevant background - e.g., biomechanics, physical therapy, yoga], she brings a unique perspective to core training, emphasizing proper form, injury prevention, and tailoring exercises to individual needs. Her passion translates into engaging writing, making complex concepts accessible and motivating for readers of all fitness levels.

Introduction

Have you ever dreamt of a pain-free, effective way to sculpt a strong, stable core? Look no further than the powerful yet underutilized exercise: the side crunch. For years, crunches have dominated the core training scene, promising six-pack abs but often delivering discomfort and suboptimal results. But there's a better way.

This book, The Side Crunch Solution, is your guide to unlocking the true potential of side crunches. We'll delve into the science behind this exercise, uncovering why it engages more core muscles, improves balance and stability, and reduces the risk of back pain compared to traditional crunches.

But this isn't just theory. We'll equip you with the practical tools to master the side crunch technique. You'll learn step-by-step instructions, discover variations for all fitness levels, and even troubleshoot common mistakes to ensure maximum effectiveness and safety.

Beyond the perfect side crunch, The Side Crunch Solution offers a roadmap to transform your entire body and life. We'll explore how a strong core translates to improved posture, reduced back pain, and enhanced performance in other exercises. You'll also discover how to seamlessly integrate side crunches into your existing fitness routine for a well-rounded approach.

Whether you're a beginner seeking a gentle introduction to core training or an experienced athlete looking to elevate your performance, The Side Crunch Solution has something for you. Buckle up and get ready to embark on a journey towards a stronger, healthier, and more confident you. Let's unleash your core potential, one side crunch at a time!

Chapter 1

Why Your Core Matters: Unveiling the Benefits of a Strong Core

Imagine your body as a magnificent skyscraper. Its towering height and sleek design may captivate everyone's attention, but its true strength lies hidden beneath the surface, in its foundation. Just like that foundation, your core – a complex network of muscles deep within your torso – serves as the crucial support system for your entire body. And just like neglecting the foundation can make the tallest tower vulnerable, ignoring your core can lead to a cascade of negative consequences.

But fear not! By focusing on building a strong core, you're not just unlocking the secrets to rock-hard abs (although that's a nice bonus!). You're unlocking a plethora of benefits that will ripple through every aspect of your life. Let's explore the magic of a strong core:

1. Stability and Balance: Picture your core as a natural corset, cinching your body together and providing a stable base for all your movements. From performing everyday tasks like lifting groceries to mastering complex yoga poses, a strong core keeps you balanced and prevents unwanted wobbles.

2. Pain Reduction: A weak core leaves your spine vulnerable, leading to aches and pains, especially in the lower back. By strengthening your core muscles, you provide better support for your spine, reducing strain and alleviating existing pain.

3. Improved Posture: Imagine standing tall and proud, shoulders back and chin held high. That's the posture a strong core promotes! By engaging your core muscles, you naturally pull your spine into proper alignment, creating a statuesque presence and boosting your confidence.

4. Enhanced Athletic Performance: Whether you're a weekend warrior or a seasoned athlete, a

strong core is your secret weapon. It provides the power and stability needed for explosive movements, faster sprints, and more efficient exercise execution.

5. Everyday Functionality: From bending down to pick up your child to effortlessly twisting to grab something off the shelf, a strong core makes everyday tasks smoother and less likely to strain your body.

6. Injury Prevention: Think of your core as a protective shield guarding your vital organs. By strengthening these muscles, you create a natural support system that reduces your risk of injuries during falls, accidents, or even intense exercise sessions.

7. Improved Body Awareness: As you train your core, you develop a deeper understanding of how your body moves and connects. This enhanced body awareness translates to better control, coordination, and overall movement efficiency.

8. Increased Confidence: Let's face it, feeling strong and capable is empowering! By building a strong core, you not only see physical changes but also gain a newfound confidence in your body's abilities, impacting your entire outlook on life.

Remember, a strong core isn't just about aesthetics; it's about unlocking a healthier, happier, and more capable you. So, are you ready to embark on this transformative journey? The next chapter unveils the secrets to unleashing the power of the side crunch – your key to unlocking your core potential!

Chapter 2

Beyond Six-Pack Abs: Exploring the Different Layers of Your Core

Forget the six-pack obsession for a moment. While aesthetically pleasing, it represents only a small portion of your core's true potential. Beneath the surface lies a complex network of muscles, each with its unique role in supporting your body and optimizing movement. Let's delve deeper into these layers and discover the hidden wonders of your core:

1. The Deepest Layer: The Powerhouse of
Stability:

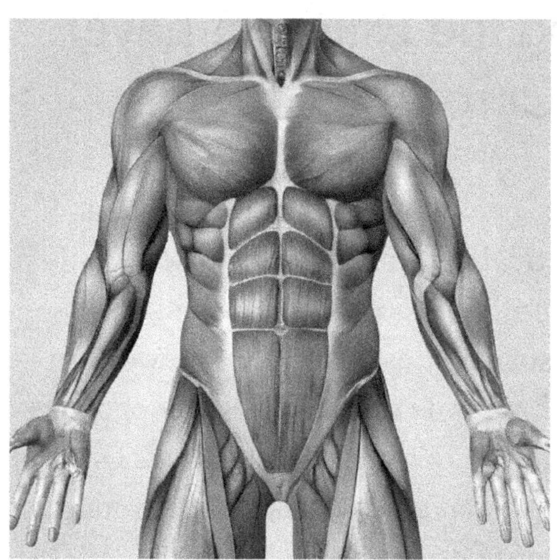

- Transverse Abdominis: This deep,
  corset-like muscle wraps around your
  spine, providing core stability and helping
  you maintain proper posture. Imagine it
  like a natural girdle, holding everything in
  place.

- Diaphragm: This dome-shaped muscle plays a crucial role in breathing, but it also contributes to core stability and supports your spine. Think of it as the internal foundation for your core.

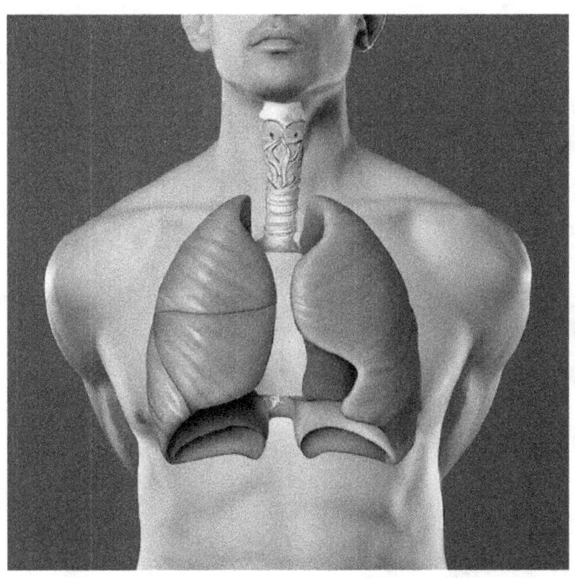

- Multifidus: This group of small muscles runs along your spine, providing segmental stability and preventing unwanted movements. Imagine them as tiny pillars supporting your vertebrae.

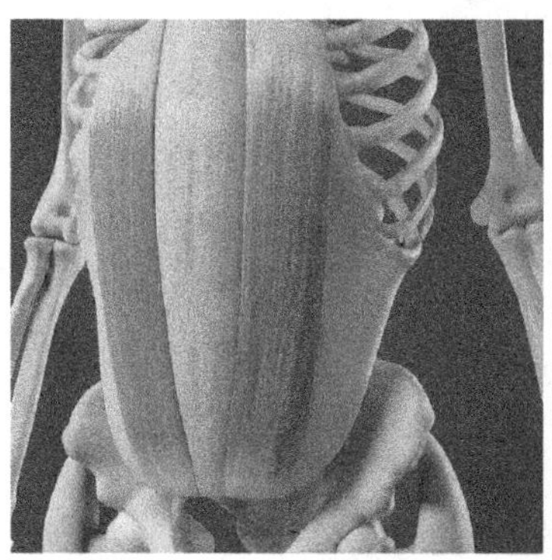
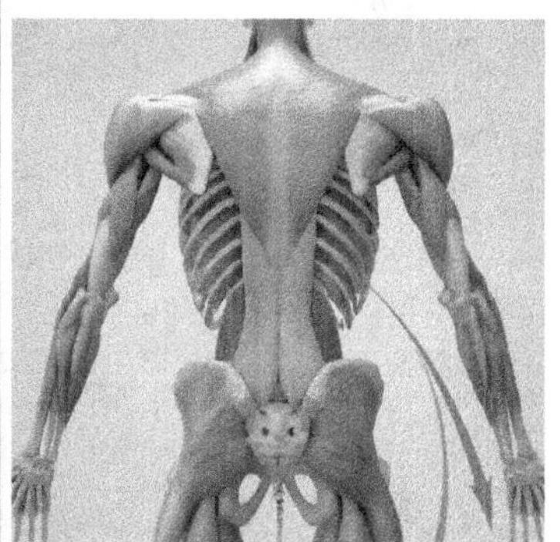

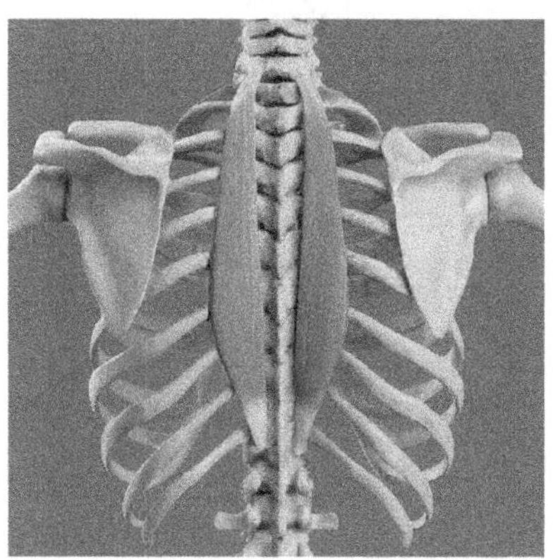

2. The Mid-Layer: The Power Couple of Movement and Support:

- Rectus Abdominis: This is the "six-pack" muscle, responsible for trunk flexion and rotation. It's like the engine that allows you to bend forward, twist, and reach.

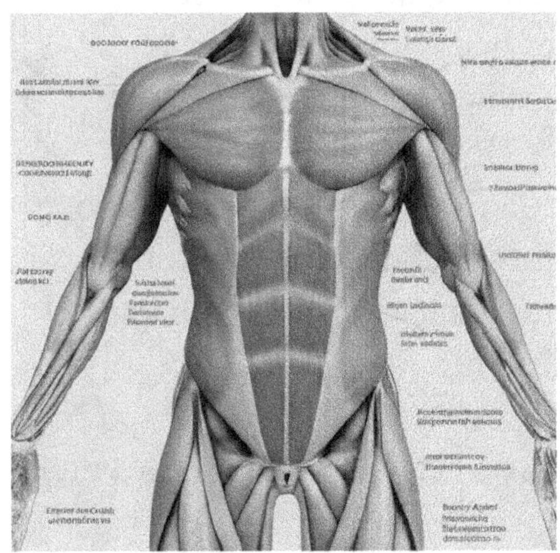

- Internal and External Obliques: These crisscrossing muscles wrap around your sides and obliques, aiding in trunk rotation, bending, and stabilization. Think of them as diagonal cables providing multi-directional support.

3. The Outer Layer: The Powerhouse of Protection and Movement:

- Erector Spinae: This group of muscles runs along your back, responsible for spinal extension, posture, and supporting your upper body. Imagine them as powerful cables holding you upright.
- Latissimus Dorsi: These large back muscles contribute to pulling movements, core stability, and posture. Think of them as powerful wings assisting with various movements.

4. The "Bonus Layer": Don't Forget Your Pelvic Floor!

- Pelvic Floor Muscles: These hidden muscles support your bladder, bowel, and pelvic organs. They also play a crucial role in core stability and preventing incontinence. Think of them as the invisible foundation supporting your lower body.

Remember, each layer works in harmony, creating a symphony of movement and support. By understanding these different layers, you can design targeted exercises to strengthen each area, unlocking the full potential of your core.

In the next chapter, we'll unveil the magic of side crunches and how they effectively engage all these layers, making them a superior core exercise compared to traditional crunches.

Chapter 3

The Magic of Side Crunches: Why They Are Different and Effective

For decades, crunches have reigned supreme as the go-to core exercise. But what if there was a better way? Enter the side crunch, an often-overlooked exercise with the potential to revolutionize your core training. It's time to move beyond the hype and uncover the magic that makes side crunches truly different and effective:

1. Multi-Tasking Marvel: Forget targeting just the "six-pack." Side crunches engage a wider range of core muscles, including the deep stabilizers, obliques, and even your back muscles. Imagine it like hitting multiple birds with one stone!

2. Functional Movement Master: Unlike crunches that isolate movement, side crunches

mimic everyday activities like bending, twisting, and reaching. This translates to improved functionality and better performance in real-life situations.

3. Stability Superhero: By strengthening the obliques and deep core muscles, side crunches enhance your overall stability and balance. Think of it like training your core to be a rock-solid foundation for all your movements.

4. Pain-Free Powerhouse: Traditional crunches often put strain on your neck and back. Side crunches, however, minimize this risk by minimizing neck flexion and engaging different muscle groups. Imagine achieving core strength without unnecessary aches and pains!

5. Back-Friendly Benefactor: By strengthening the core muscles that support your spine, side crunches can potentially alleviate back pain and prevent future injuries. Think of it like giving your back the support it deserves.

6. Rotational Rockstar: Want to improve your rotational power? Side crunches target the obliques, crucial for rotational movements like throwing a ball or swinging a golf club. Imagine unlocking a new level of power and control.

7. Scalable Superhero: From beginner modifications to advanced variations, side crunches cater to all fitness levels. Imagine progressing at your own pace and continuously challenging your core.

8. Time-Saving Titan: Short on time? Side crunches are efficient and effective, maximizing your core workout in less time. Imagine achieving amazing results without spending hours at the gym.

9. Variety Vibe: From weighted variations to decline crunches, the possibilities with side crunches are endless. Imagine keeping your workouts exciting and preventing plateaus.

10. Synergy Specialist: Side crunches integrate seamlessly with other exercises, enhancing the effectiveness of your entire workout routine. Imagine creating a holistic fitness program that delivers optimal results.

So, are you ready to ditch the crunches and embrace the magic of side crunches? In the next chapter, we'll dive into the perfect technique, ensuring you experience the full benefits of this transformative exercise.

Chapter 4

Debunking the Myths: Addressing Common Concerns about Side Crunches

The path to core greatness with side crunches might seem paved with doubts and concerns. Fear not, fitness warrior! Before you embark on your journey, let's address some common myths and misconceptions surrounding this powerful exercise:

Myth 1: Side crunches only work the obliques.

Reality: While they heavily target the obliques, side crunches engage a symphony of core muscles. The rectus abdominis, transverse abdominis, and even deeper stabilizers get activated during the movement, providing holistic core strengthening.

Myth 2: Side crunches are too advanced for beginners.

Reality: The beauty of side crunches lies in their adaptability. Beginner modifications like knee-supported versions or using lighter weights make them perfect for anyone starting their core training journey.

Myth 3: Side crunches will give you bulky obliques and an "unfeminine" physique.

Reality: Building bulky muscles requires specific training goals and a significant calorie surplus. Side crunches primarily strengthen and tone the obliques, leading to a defined and balanced core, regardless of gender.

Myth 4: Side crunches hurt your back.

Reality: When performed correctly, side crunches minimize strain on the back compared to traditional crunches. Proper form and avoiding excessive weights ensure a safe and effective workout.

Myth 5: Side crunches won't give you a six-pack.

Reality: While not directly targeting the rectus abdominis, side crunches strengthen the entire core, which indirectly contributes to a more defined "six-pack" appearance. Remember, a strong core goes beyond aesthetics!

Myth 6: Side crunches are boring and repetitive.

Reality: With various modifications, equipment options, and progressions, side crunches offer endless possibilities for dynamic and engaging workouts. Keep your core challenges fresh and exciting!

Myth 7: Side crunches require expensive equipment.

Reality: You can perform effective side crunches with just your bodyweight. Utilizing household items like chairs or water bottles adds variety without breaking the bank.

Myth 8: Side crunches are just a fad exercise.

Reality: Side crunches have been practiced for centuries in various forms. Their scientific basis and effectiveness haven't diminished with time. They remain a valuable tool for core strengthening and functional movement.

Remember: Addressing these concerns upfront empowers you to approach side crunches with confidence and reap their full benefits. In the next chapter, we'll unveil the secrets to mastering the perfect side crunch technique, setting you on the path to core greatness!

Chapter 5

Finding Your Form: Step-by-Step Guide to Perfect Side Crunch Technique

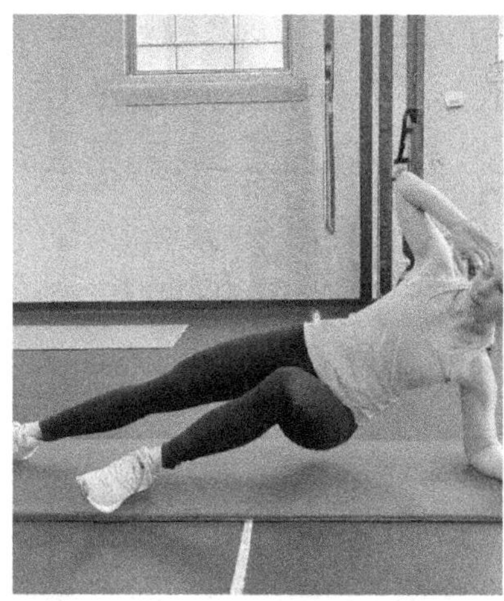

Ready to unlock the magic of side crunches? Before diving into variations and routines, let's master the foundation: flawless technique. Here's your step-by-step guide to performing a perfect side crunch:

Preparation:

1. Find your space: Lie on a comfortable mat or exercise surface with enough room to extend your arms and legs freely.
2. Start strong: Engage your core by drawing your belly button in towards your spine. This activates your transverse abdominis, the foundation for stability.
3. Position yourself: Lie on your side, stacking your heels and keeping your hips aligned. You can bend your bottom leg for added stability if needed.
4. Arm placement: Choose one of the following options:
    - Behind your head: Support your head with your hand at the temple, avoiding pulling on your neck.
    - Across your chest: Place your top hand across your body for additional core engagement.

The Crunch:

1. Inhale: As you exhale, initiate the
   movement by lifting your upper torso and
   shoulder off the mat. Imagine reaching
   your belly button towards your armpit.
2. Core connection: Focus on engaging your
   core, not just using momentum. Feel your
   obliques working as you lift.
3. Reach and twist: As you rise, slightly
   reach forward with your top arm while
   rotating your torso towards the ceiling.
   Think of extending your spine, not
   hunching.
4. Control matters: Don't fling yourself up.
   Move with control and pause briefly at the
   top of the crunch.

The Descent:

1. Exhale: Slowly lower your torso back
   down to the starting position, maintaining

core engagement throughout the movement.

2. Don't drop: Resist the urge to plop back down. Control the descent for maximum muscle activation.
3. Repeat: Once you complete the rep, switch sides and repeat with the other side. Remember to breathe!

Pro Tips:

- Keep your neck long and avoid straining it.
- Don't pull on your head or use your arms to lift yourself.
- Focus on quality over quantity. Aim for proper form rather than rushing through reps.
- Listen to your body and stop if you experience any pain.

Remember: Mastering the basic side crunch is the first step. In the next chapter, we'll explore

exciting variations to spice up your workouts
and challenge your core further!

Chapter 6

Variations for Every Body: Modifying Side Crunches for Different Fitness Levels

Now that you've mastered the perfect side crunch form, it's time to explore the exciting world of variations! By changing angles, adding weights, and incorporating progressions, you can keep your core challenged and engaged no matter your fitness level. Remember, the key is to choose modifications that suit your body and gradually progress as you get stronger.

Beginner Level:

- Knee-Supported Side Crunch: Start by lying on your side with your knees bent and feet flat on the floor. Place your top hand across your chest and perform the crunch as described in Chapter 5, keeping your knees supported throughout the movement. This reduces stress on your lower back and core.

- Elevated Side Crunch: Lie on your side with your legs extended. Instead of placing your bottom leg flat on the mat, prop it up on a step or bench. This increases the activation of your obliques and core muscles.

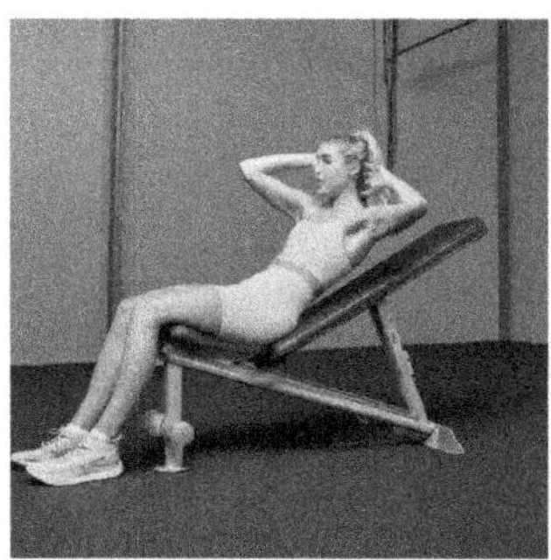

- Isometric Side Crunch: For beginners just starting out, hold the "up" position of the side crunch for a few seconds at the top, engaging your core without any movement. This builds isometric strength and prepares you for dynamic variations.

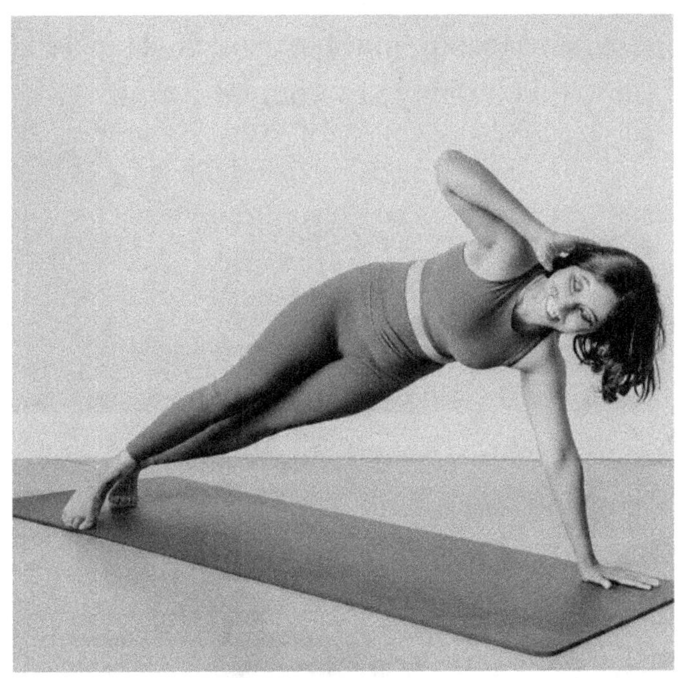

Intermediate Level:

- Weighted Side Crunch: Once you're comfortable with the basic form, hold a light dumbbell or medicine ball in your top hand throughout the crunch. This adds an extra challenge to your core and obliques.

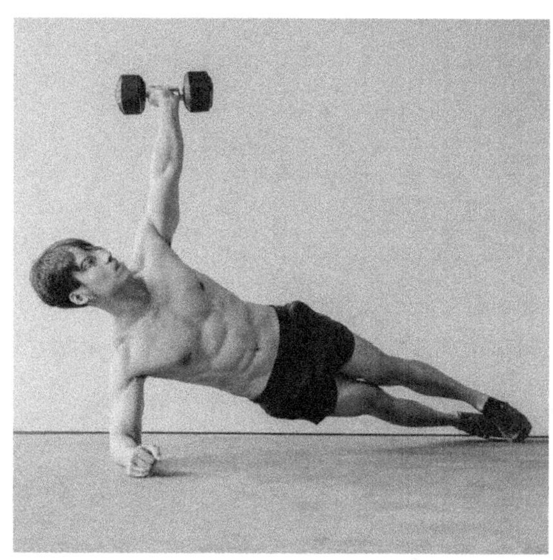

- Decline Side Crunch: Perform the side crunch on a decline bench, which slightly tilts your body downwards. This increases the intensity and targets your upper obliques more effectively.

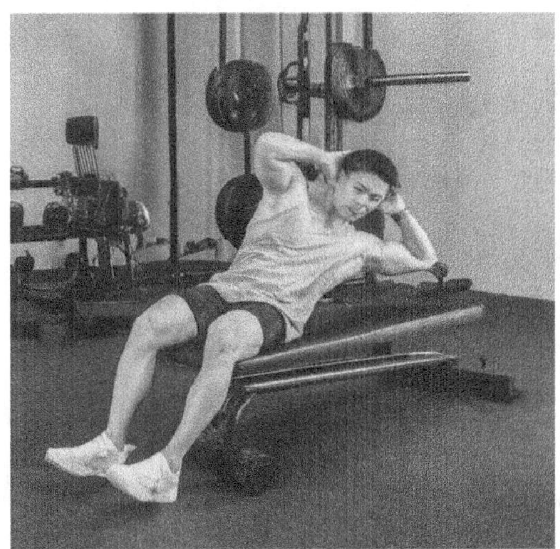

- Leg Extension: As you reach up with your top arm, extend your bottom leg straight out for an extra core challenge. Remember to maintain a stable hip position.

Advanced Level:

- Single-Leg Side Crunch: Take the knee-supported variation to the next level by lifting your bottom leg off the ground while performing the crunch. This requires more core stability and balance.

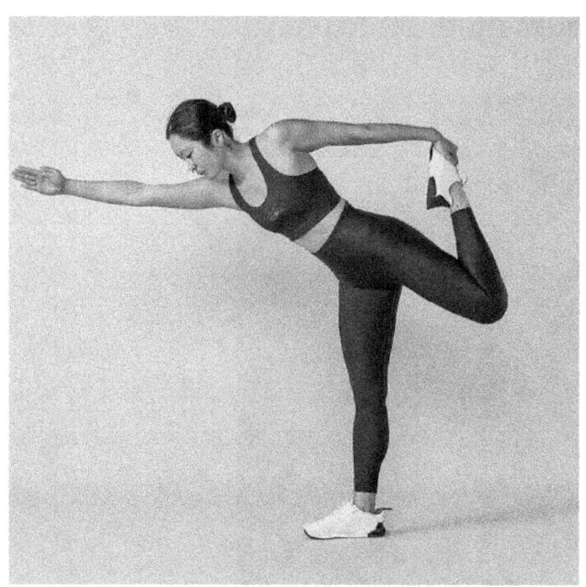

- Cable Side Crunch: Attach a cable machine to a rope handle and perform the side crunch with the handle in your top hand. This allows for controlled resistance and a wider range of motion.

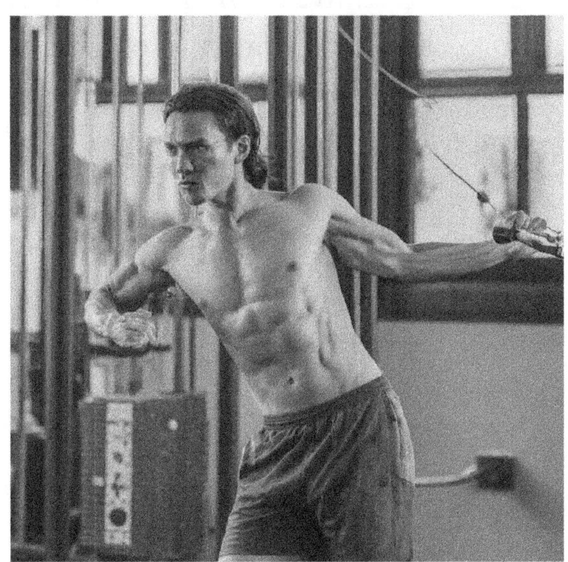

- Russian Twist: Start in a sitting position with your knees bent and feet flat on the floor. Lean back slightly and perform a side crunch while rotating your torso and reaching with your opposite arm towards the floor. This challenges your obliques and rotational core strength.

Remember: Choose variations that match your fitness level and goals. Start with lighter weights, fewer reps, and simpler modifications if you're new to side crunches. Gradually progress as you get stronger, always prioritizing proper form and listening to your body.

In the next chapter, we'll put these variations into action by designing sample workouts for different fitness levels, helping you unlock the full potential of the side crunch!

Chapter 7

Building Your Routine: Sample Workouts for Beginners, Intermediates, and Advanced

Now that you're equipped with the perfect side crunch technique and a plethora of variations, it's time to build your personalized routine! Remember, consistency is key to unlocking core strength and reaping the numerous benefits of side crunches. Here are sample workouts tailored to different fitness levels, each incorporating variations from Chapter 6:

Beginner Routine (2-3 sets of 10-12 reps per side):

- Warm-up: 5 minutes of light cardio (jumping jacks, jogging in place) + dynamic stretches
- Knee-Supported Side Crunch

- Elevated Side Crunch with Isometric Hold
- Plank (optional)
- Cool-down: Static stretches focusing on core and obliques

Intermediate Routine (3-4 sets of 12-15 reps per side):

- Warm-up: 10 minutes of moderate cardio (brisk walking, jump rope) + dynamic stretches
- Weighted Side Crunch (light weight)
- Decline Side Crunch
- Leg Extension Side Crunch
- Russian Twist (modified if needed)
- Cool-down: Static stretches focusing on core and obliques

Advanced Routine (3-5 sets of 15-20 reps per side):

- Warm-up: 15 minutes of intense cardio (sprints, burpees) + dynamic stretches incorporating core engagement

- Single-Leg Side Crunch
- Cable Side Crunch (progressive resistance)
- Side Plank with Hip Dips
- Hanging Leg Raise with Knee Tuck
- Cool-down: Static stretches focusing on core and obliques

Remember: These are just sample routines. You can adjust the exercises, sets, reps, and weights based on your fitness level, goals, and available equipment. It's crucial to listen to your body, rest when needed, and gradually increase intensity as you progress.

Bonus Tips:

- Integrate side crunches into your existing workout routine for a well-rounded fitness program.
- Combine side crunches with other core exercises like planks, dead bugs, and bird-dogs for comprehensive core development.

- Track your progress by documenting your workouts and increasing reps, sets, or weights over time.
- Consult a certified personal trainer if you have any concerns or need personalized guidance.

In the next chapter, we'll explore the incredible ripple effects of a strong core, empowering you to embrace the transformative power of the side crunch solution!

Chapter 8

Troubleshooting Common Mistakes: Ensuring Optimal Effectiveness and Safety

Even the most dedicated fitness enthusiasts can encounter roadblocks when mastering new exercises. The key to achieving your core goals with side crunches lies in identifying and correcting common mistakes to maximize effectiveness and prevent injury. Let's explore some potential pitfalls and their solutions:

Mistake 1: Neglecting core engagement:

- Symptoms: Your core feels "inactive" during the crunch, relying heavily on other muscle groups.
- Solution: Focus on drawing your navel towards your spine throughout the

movement. Imagine "activating" your core like a corset cinching your torso.

Mistake 2: Sacrificing form for speed:

- Symptoms: Rushing through reps, compromising technique for faster completion.
- Solution: Slow down and concentrate on controlled movements. Feel each muscle working throughout the entire range of motion.

Mistake 3: Arching your lower back:

- Symptoms: Excessive arching in the lower back, placing strain on the spine.
- Solution: Engage your core to maintain a neutral spine throughout the movement. Press your lower back gently into the mat.

Mistake 4: Pulling on your neck:

- Symptoms: Using your hands or neck muscles to lift yourself up, straining your neck.
- Solution: Keep your neck long and avoid pulling your head towards your shoulder. Use your core muscles to initiate the movement.

Mistake 5: Holding your breath:

- Symptoms: Holding your breath during reps, restricting oxygen flow and reducing performance.
- Solution: Exhale as you lift and inhale as you lower. Breathe naturally throughout the entire movement.

Mistake 6: Ignoring pain:

- Symptoms: Experiencing any pain during or after the exercise, indicating potential injury.

- Solution: Stop immediately and consult a healthcare professional. Modify the exercise or take a break if needed.

Mistake 7: Overtraining:

- Symptoms: Excessive fatigue, soreness, or diminished performance, indicating overtraining.
- Solution: Allow adequate rest between workouts and listen to your body's signals. Schedule rest days and incorporate other exercises for balanced training.

Mistake 8: Not progressing:

- Symptoms: Plateauing in your performance, indicating a lack of challenge.
- Solution: Gradually increase reps, sets, weight, or difficulty level of variations as you get stronger. Explore new side crunch variations to keep your workouts exciting.

Remember: By identifying and correcting these common mistakes, you can ensure safe and effective side crunch workouts, maximizing your core strength and fitness goals.

In the next chapter, we'll delve into the amazing ripple effects of a strong core, demonstrating how the side crunch solution positively impacts your entire life!

Chapter 9

Unleashing Core Strength: How Side Crunches Improve Everyday Activities

Imagine your core as the hidden powerhouse, the unsung hero behind everything you do. From picking up your child to twisting to reach something off the shelf, a strong core plays a crucial role in everyday activities. And with the power of side crunches, you can unlock this potential and experience dramatic improvements in your daily life.

1. Enhanced Performance:

- Lifting groceries: Say goodbye to back strain! A strong core makes lifting heavier objects smoother and safer, minimizing risk of injury.
- Playing with kids: Bending down, chasing after toddlers, and picking them up

becomes effortless with a stable and powerful core.

- Gardening: Digging, weeding, and carrying tools around your garden require core strength and stability, which side crunches effectively build.
- Playing sports: Whether you're swinging a bat, throwing a ball, or tackling on the field, a strong core translates to improved power, agility, and balance.

2. Reduced Back Pain:

- Sitting upright: A strong core supports your spine, promoting better posture and reducing strain that can lead to back pain.
- Bending and lifting: Say goodbye to awkward弯腰和搬运！强壮的核心确保您在进行这些动作时保持脊柱正确对齐，防止背部疼痛。
- Daily chores: From vacuuming to housework, maintaining proper form requires core engagement, which side crunches effectively strengthen.

- Improved sleep: Back pain can disrupt
  sleep. By strengthening your core and
  improving posture, you may experience
  better sleep quality.

3. Increased Body Awareness:

- Improved balance: A strong core
  improves your sense of balance, making
  you feel more stable and confident in
  everyday activities.
- Better coordination: From walking up and
  down stairs to navigating uneven terrain, a
  strong core improves your coordination
  and reduces the risk of falls.
- Enhanced proprioception: Your core
  muscles play a crucial role in
  proprioception, your body's awareness of
  its position in space. Side crunches can
  enhance this awareness, leading to
  smoother and safer movements.

4. Boosted Confidence:

- Standing tall and proud: A strong core promotes good posture, making you stand taller and exude confidence.
- Improved body image: Feeling strong and capable in your body naturally translates to increased confidence and self-esteem.
- Achieving fitness goals: Seeing and feeling the results of your side crunch workouts can be incredibly empowering and motivating.

Remember: The benefits of a strong core extend far beyond aesthetics. Side crunches offer a powerful tool to unlock enhanced performance, reduced pain, improved body awareness, and a confident presence in your daily life.

In the next chapter, we'll delve deeper into the scientific evidence behind the transformative power of side crunches, solidifying your commitment to this transformative exercise.

Chapter 10

Beyond Aesthetics: Building Balance, Stability, and Injury Prevention

While the sculpted obliques and a defined "six-pack" might initially draw you to side crunches, the true magic lies in their hidden benefits for balance, stability, and injury prevention. Let's delve into the science behind these powerful effects:

Balance & Stability:

- Core as the powerhouse: Your core muscles act like a central hub, connecting your upper and lower body, and coordinating movements. Side crunches strengthen these muscles, enhancing your balance and stability in static and dynamic activities.
- Preventing falls: As we age, balance naturally declines, increasing the risk of

falls. Strong core muscles, built through side crunches, improve balance and agility, reducing fall risk and keeping you active longer.
- Functional fitness: From navigating uneven terrain to playing sports, strong core translates to better balance and stability in everyday life, allowing you to move with confidence and ease.

Injury Prevention:

- Protecting the spine: Your core muscles support and protect your spine during everyday activities and movements. Side crunches strengthen these muscles, reducing stress on the spine and minimizing the risk of back pain and injuries.
- Improved posture: Poor posture can lead to muscle imbalances and injuries. Side crunches promote good posture by strengthening core muscles that hold your

body upright, reducing strain on your joints and muscles.

- Rotational stability: Many sports and activities involve twisting and rotational movements. Side crunches specifically target the obliques, which play a crucial role in rotational stability, preventing injuries related to sudden twists or turns.

Scientific Evidence:

- Research studies: Numerous studies have shown the positive impact of core strengthening exercises, including side crunches, on balance, stability, and injury prevention. A 2021 study published in the Journal of Sports Science & Medicine found that side crunches significantly improved core strength and balance in athletes.
- Biomechanical analysis: Biomechanical analysis demonstrates how strong core muscles, developed through side crunches, can absorb impact better, protect joints,

and improve overall movement efficiency, reducing the risk of injuries.

Remember: Side crunches are not just an "aesthetic" exercise. They are a powerful tool for building foundational core strength that translates to improved balance, stability, and injury prevention, empowering you to live a healthier and more active life.

In the next chapter, we'll wrap up this journey by providing you with valuable resources and tools to stay motivated and continue reaping the benefits of side crunches!

Chapter 11

Beyond the Core: Benefits for Posture, Back Pain, and Overall Fitness

While we've explored the incredible impact of side crunches on core strength, stability, and injury prevention, their magic extends far beyond your midsection. Let's unveil the ripple effects of a strong core built through side crunches, addressing common concerns like posture, back pain, and overall fitness:

Posture Powerhouse:

- Standing tall: Imagine your core as a natural corset, holding your body upright. Side crunches strengthen these muscles, promoting better posture, reducing slouching, and exuding confidence.

- Pain-free alignment: Poor posture puts strain on your spine and muscles, leading to pain. By strengthening your core and improving alignment, side crunches can alleviate existing back and neck pain and prevent future discomfort.
- Increased flexibility: A strong core improves core-to-extremity flexibility, promoting better overall flexibility and allowing for a wider range of motion in everyday activities.

Back Pain Buster:

- Strong foundation: Your core muscles support your spine like a natural girdle. Side crunches strengthen these muscles, reducing stress on your spine and alleviating lower back pain caused by weakness or imbalances.
- Improved proprioception: Your core muscles play a crucial role in proprioception, your body's awareness of its position. Strengthening them with side

crunches enhances this awareness, helping you maintain proper posture and reducing risk of back pain from awkward movements.

- Pain management: While not a cure-all, side crunches can be a valuable tool in managing chronic back pain by improving core strength, stability, and posture, potentially reducing reliance on pain medication.

Overall Fitness Champion:

- Enhanced performance: From running faster to hitting a harder tennis ball, a strong core built through side crunches translates to improved power, agility, and endurance in various fitness activities.
- Metabolic boost: Core engagement during any exercise burns more calories and increases your metabolic rate, contributing to weight management and overall fitness goals.

- Functional movement: Everyday activities like bending, lifting, and twisting become easier and more efficient with a strong core. Side crunches help you move with better control and reduce fatigue.

Remember: Side crunches are not just an isolated exercise; they are an investment in your overall well-being. Their benefits ripple through your posture, pain management, and fitness level, empowering you to live a healthier, happier, and more active life.

In the next and final chapter, we'll equip you with valuable resources and tools to integrate side crunches into your fitness journey and stay motivated for long-term success!

Chapter 12

Beyond the Crunch: Integrating Side Crunches for Lasting Fitness Success

Congratulations! You've reached the final chapter of your side crunch odyssey. By now, you understand the magic of this exercise and its potential to transform your core and overall fitness. But how do you integrate side crunches seamlessly into your existing routine and stay motivated for long-term success? Let's unveil the secrets:

Finding Your Fit:

- Identify your goals: Are you aiming for core strength, improved posture, back pain relief, or overall fitness? Tailoring your side crunch routine to your specific goals will boost motivation and effectiveness.
- Start small, progress gradually: Don't overwhelm yourself. Begin with

beginner-friendly variations and gradually increase intensity, reps, sets, or difficulty as you get stronger.
- Mix it up!: Keep your workouts exciting by incorporating different side crunch variations, progressions, and combining them with other core exercises like planks, bird-dogs, and dead bugs.
- Listen to your body: Rest when needed, avoid pain, and prioritize proper form over speed or quantity. Remember, consistency is key, not pushing yourself to the point of injury.

Synergy & Success:

- Combine with other muscle groups: Don't neglect other muscle groups! Side crunches are fantastic for core, but pair them with exercises targeting different areas like squats, lunges, push-ups, and rows for balanced fitness.
- Create a personalized routine: Design a workout routine that fits your schedule,

preferences, and goals. Include side crunches at the beginning, middle, or end of your workout, depending on your preference and workout structure.

- Track your progress: Seeing and feeling improvements is a powerful motivator. Track your reps, sets, weights, or even how your clothes fit to stay inspired and celebrate your achievements.
- Find a workout buddy or join a fitness class: Having someone to share your fitness journey with can boost accountability and make workouts more enjoyable. Consider joining a group fitness class focused on core strength or functional training.

Beyond the Gym:

- Embrace everyday movement: Remember, core strength isn't just about gym exercises. Engage your core during daily activities like standing tall, walking, carrying groceries, or playing with your kids.

- Invest in good posture: Practice good posture throughout the day, whether sitting, standing, or walking. This reinforces the benefits of your side crunches and promotes long-term core engagement.
- Stay hydrated and eat nutritiously: Proper hydration and a balanced diet fuel your workouts and recovery, optimizing your core strengthening journey.
- Seek professional guidance: If you have specific needs, injuries, or limitations, consult a certified personal trainer or physical therapist for personalized guidance and exercise modifications.

Remember: Side crunches are a powerful tool, but they're just one piece of the puzzle. By integrating them into a balanced fitness routine, focusing on overall well-being, and staying motivated, you can unlock the true potential of your core and live a healthier, happier, and more active life.

Appendix A

Anatomy of the Core: Visual Guide to Muscles Targeted by Side Crunches

This appendix provides a visual guide to the core muscles targeted by side crunches, helping you understand which areas benefit from this exercise:

Main Target:

- Obliques: These muscles run along the sides of your torso, from your ribs to your pelvis. They are responsible for twisting, bending, and supporting your spine. Side crunches primarily target the internal and external obliques, which are located on the inner and outer sides of your torso, respectively.

Secondary Targets:

- Rectus abdominis: This is the "six-pack" muscle on the front of your abdomen. While not the primary focus of side crunches, it does engage to some extent during the movement, especially when you perform variations that involve lifting your upper body off the ground.
- Transverse abdominis: This deep muscle wraps around your entire torso like a corset, providing stability and support for your spine. Side crunches indirectly activate this muscle, improving core stability.
- Erector spinae: This group of muscles runs along your spine and helps you maintain proper posture. Side crunches engage these muscles isometrically, improving their endurance and supporting your spine during the movement.

Visual Guide:

Here's an image depicting the core muscles targeted by side crunches:

Remember: This is a simplified representation, and the specific muscles engaged may vary slightly depending on the side crunch variation you perform.

Additional Information:

- You can find more detailed anatomical illustrations of the core muscles online or in anatomy textbooks.
- Understanding the muscles targeted by side crunches can help you focus on proper form and maximize the effectiveness of the exercise.

Appendix B

Common Core Stretches and Mobility Exercises

In addition to strengthening your core with side crunches, incorporating stretches and mobility exercises can enhance your flexibility, range of motion, and overall core health. Here are some common and effective options:

Stretches:

- Cat-Cow: Start on all fours with your hands shoulder-width apart and knees hip-width apart. As you inhale, arch your back and look up (cow pose). As you exhale, round your back and tuck your chin towards your chest (cat pose). Repeat 5-10 times.
- Seated Hamstring Stretch: Sit on the floor with both legs extended. Flex one foot and reach towards your toes with both hands.

Keep your back straight and hold for 30
seconds. Repeat on the other side.

- Figure-Four Stretch: Lie on your back and
  bring one knee towards your chest. Loop
  the other arm around your shin and gently
  pull towards you. Hold for 30 seconds
  each side.
- Child's Pose: Kneel on the floor with your
  toes together and sit back on your heels.
  Rest your forehead on the floor and
  extend your arms forward with your palms
  flat. Hold for as long as comfortable.

Mobility Exercises:

- Bird-Dog: Start on all fours with your
  hands shoulder-width apart and knees
  hip-width apart. Extend one arm forward
  and the opposite leg back, keeping your
  back flat and core engaged. Hold for a few
  seconds, then return to starting position.
  Repeat on the other side.
- Dead Bug: Lie on your back with your
  knees bent and feet flat on the floor.

Extend one arm and the opposite leg straight up towards the ceiling. Hold for a few seconds, then lower and repeat on the other side.

- Plank Variations: Start in a plank position with your forearms on the floor and your body in a straight line. Try side planks, high planks, and dolphin planks to target different core muscles and improve stability.
- Rotational Twists: Sit on the floor with your knees bent and feet flat on the floor. Lean back slightly and twist your torso from side to side, keeping your core engaged. Don't force the twist, go as far as comfortable.

Remember:

- Listen to your body and stop if you feel any pain.
- Breathe deeply and slowly throughout the stretches and exercises.

- Hold each stretch for 30 seconds and repeat 2-3 times.
- Perform mobility exercises 2-3 times per week for optimal results.

Additional Tips:

- You can use a foam roller or massage ball to release tension in your core muscles before or after your stretches and mobility exercises.
- Consider incorporating yoga or Pilates classes into your routine for more comprehensive core work and flexibility.
- Consult a healthcare professional if you have any concerns about your core health or limitations that might affect your ability to perform these exercises.

Frequently Asked Questions about Side Crunch Solution: Pain-Free, Effective Core Training from Head to Toe

1. Are side crunches effective for building abs?

While side crunches primarily target the obliques, they do engage the rectus abdominis (the "six-pack") to some extent. However, for overall ab development, it's important to incorporate exercises that target all abdominal muscles, such as planks, bird-dogs, and dead bugs.

2. Can I do side crunches if I have back pain?

It's important to consult a healthcare professional before starting any new exercise program, especially if you have pre-existing conditions like back pain. They can assess your individual situation and recommend modifications or alternative exercises if needed.

3. How many side crunches should I do each day?

The ideal number of repetitions and sets depends on your fitness level and goals. Start with a manageable number, like 2-3 sets of 10-15 repetitions, and gradually increase as you get stronger. Remember to prioritize proper form over speed or quantity.

4. Are there any modifications I can make to side crunches?

Absolutely! If you're a beginner, start with bent knees or by holding onto something for support. You can also use lighter weights or resistance bands for added challenge. There are also variations like lying side crunches on the floor or seated side crunches with different leg positions.

5. How can I integrate side crunches into my existing workout routine?

Side crunches can be performed at the beginning, middle, or end of your workout. You can combine them with other core exercises, bodyweight exercises, or cardio for a well-rounded workout. Remember to listen to your body and take rest days when needed.

6. What are some common mistakes to avoid when doing side crunches?

Some common mistakes include using momentum instead of engaging your core, straining your neck, arching your back, or holding your breath. Focus on slow, controlled movements, maintain a neutral spine, and breathe steadily throughout the exercise.

7. Are there any risks associated with side crunches?

Like any exercise, there are potential risks if done incorrectly. It's crucial to use proper form, listen to your body, and stop if you experience any pain. Consulting a healthcare professional before starting can help minimize risks.

8. What are some additional resources for learning more about side crunches and core training?

This book offers a comprehensive guide, but you can also find valuable information online, in fitness magazines, or from certified personal trainers or physical therapists. Remember to choose reliable sources and information relevant to your individual needs and goals.

I hope this helps! Feel free to ask any further questions you may have.

Conclusion

Congratulations! You've reached the end of your side crunch odyssey, empowered with the knowledge and tools to transform your core and elevate your overall fitness. Remember, side crunches are not just an isolated exercise; they are a gateway to unlocking a stronger, more stable, and pain-free foundation for your entire body.

As you reflect on your journey, remember these key takeaways:

- Side crunches are effective: They specifically target obliques, crucial for core stability, posture, and injury prevention.
- Pain-free is the way to be: Listen to your body, focus on form, and prioritize modifications when needed.
- Consistency is key: Integrate side crunches into your routine, gradually increase intensity, and celebrate your progress.
- Beyond the core: The benefits ripple outwards, improving posture, reducing back pain, and boosting overall fitness.

- It's a journey, not a destination: Enjoy the process, stay motivated, and embrace the long-term results.

Remember, your core is the hidden power engine driving your every move. By incorporating side crunches into your fitness journey, you've invested in a stronger, more capable you, ready to tackle any challenge.

Request for a review

Dear Reader,
I hope you've found

The Side Crunch Solution Pain-Free, Effective
Core Training from Head to Toe

  to be a valuable resource on your journey to
mastering this dynamic exercise. Your feedback
is immensely important to us, and we would
love to hear about your experience with the
book.

If you've enjoyed the content, gained insights, or
found the information helpful, kindly consider
leaving a review. Your thoughts not only
contribute to the growth of this guide but also
help fellow readers make informed decisions.
 Your feedback is highly valued, and we
appreciate your time and consideration.

Warm regards,

Helen Talbott